I0423887

The Sweet Side of the Stinking Rose

HOW TO USE GARLIC TO FEEL GOOD AND
LIVE LONGER

Valerie B. Lull

Copyright © 2016 by Valerie B. Lull.

All rights reserved. No part of this publication may be reproduced, distributed or transmitted in any form or by any means, including photocopying, recording, or other electronic or mechanical methods, without the prior written permission of the publisher, except in the case of brief quotations embodied in critical reviews and certain other noncommercial uses permitted by copyright law.

The information contained in this book is not intended to replace professional medical advice. Any use of the information in this book is at the reader's discretion. The author and publisher specifically disclaim any and all liability arising directly or indirectly from the use or application of any information contained in this book. It is intended for educational purposes only. A health-care professional should be consulted about your specific situation.

The Sweet Side of the Stinking Rose / Valerie B. Lull. —1st ed.
ISBN 978-1533091222

Contents

To my good friends Louise Langley, Shirley Cody and Maija Yegge, who encouraged me to follow my dream.

Why I Wrote This Book

Why write a book on garlic? Why not? In my herbal studies I have found that garlic is one of the mainstays in the herbalist's toolbox. It is useful for just about everything and it is readily available.

I find the study of integrative medicine fascinating. I got interested in anti-aging or at least slowing down the aging process, around the age of 45. I was feeling tired and run down and had developed diabetes. I had also been working in mental health for 12 years. I was ready for a career change and I chose herbal studies. I found if fascinating. So, I went to herb school to get my diploma as a master herbalist. Since then I haven't looked back and it gets more and more interesting as each day passes.

My first book was about *Ten Healthy Teas.* My second book was *Ten Spices for Health and Longevity.* This book is about garlic. There is so much out there for the herbalist to learn. There are still thousands of plants that we don't know anything about.

Plant medicine was man's first medicine and goes back for millenniums. Modern drugs have only been with us about 200 years. Herbal medicine was man's first medicine and the only medicine he had. Herbal medicine has stood the test of time.

My goal is to help people find simple ways to stay healthy and live longer. As you continue your journey I hope you find vibrant health and happiness. – Valerie Lull

CHAPTER 1

Introduction and folklore

Latin Name: *Allium Sativum*

Family: *Liliaceae*

Common Name: *Poor Man's Treacle*

I believe garlic is one of the most versatile of all the herbs. I like garlic because it is readily available at the local supermarket, it is very inexpensive, it has multiple uses, and it works.

Garlic's scientific name is *Allium sativum*, which comes from the Latin. Allium was the Latin name for garlic and sativum means cultivated. Allium describes a group of plants which include onions, leeks, shallots, and chives.

Historically garlic was called Poor Man's Treacle because people thought it counteracted poison in animals. Garlic has been studied extensively for its health benefits, and Garlic is one of the most studied of all herbs.

Garlic is a well-known herb. People use it all the time, but it should not be taken to excess. Some folks eat a few raw cloves every day. Most people either love garlic, or they hate it.

One of the reasons people don't like garlic is the odor. It comes from a chemical called allicin which is in garlic. If you are one of the people who do not like the odor, there are many garlic products on the market that give you the benefits of garlic without the odor.

Some folks like the smell and taste of garlic. It is used extensively in cooking, and Garlic tea with a little cayenne or chicken bouillon added to it is helpful for a sore throat or stuffed up sinuses.

Garlic has a long and colorful history. Garlic is thought to have originated in northwestern Asia. The ancients believed that garlic gave you strength. According to folklore, garlic was fed to the Hebrew slaves in Egypt to strengthen them. Clay figures of Garlic were found in Tutankhamen's tomb. Garlic is mentioned in the Bible and the Talmud.

The Chinese used garlic for centuries. They used it for heart attacks and circulatory problems. The ancient Greeks and Romans used garlic. Hippocrates, the father of medicine, prescribed garlic for ailments such as leprosy, wounds, digestive complaints, cancerous tumors, and heart problems.

Galen and Dioscorides used it for common disorders like poor digestion and parasites. The ancients believed that Garlic had an effect on the immune system. Both Romans and Greeks used garlic in wartime for their soldiers[1].

Garlic is legendary for repelling vampires, and garlic was used to keep away evil spirits. In the middle ages, it was used in an attempt to ward off the plague.

There was a medieval doctor by the name of Bald in A.D. 900 in England. He used garlic as a remedy for illness. Later garlic fell out of favor and was disliked by the English. Shakespeare refers to garlic as an aphrodisiac. Culpepper, an herbalist from 17th century England refers to the offensiveness of the garlic smell on the breath.

Historically the Arab doctors like Avicenna used garlic. The medieval medical school at Salerno, Italy used garlic. St. Hildegard of Bremen refers to the medicinal use of garlic in her writings.

The London College of Physicians in 1649 used garlic as an antidote to bites from venomous beasts. They also believed garlic was good for disorders of the urinary tract and the bowels. Garlic was considered to be an antidote to the bubonic plague of the 17th century.

The Chinese used garlic for worms. They used Garlic for animals. They used it for people as a preventive of influenza. Garlic was and still is used extensively in Eastern Europe. The Russians use a head of garlic with a

---

[1]http://www.whfoods.com/genpage.php?tname=foodspice&dbid=60

cup of milk for dysentery, seizures and threadworms. In the new world, garlic was introduced by the explorers from Europe.

In 1858, Louis Pasteur studied garlic and documented its antibacterial properties.

In both World War I and World War II when there were shortages of medicines, British army medics made a wash of it that they used in treating wounds. The Russians used garlic extensively on the battlefield and garlic won the title of "Russian Penicillin".

Albert Schweitzer used garlic and was aware of its antibacterial and antifungal properties. He used it to treat typhus and cholera.

For centuries, the people in northern Europe associated garlic with the Mediterranean countries and suggested that they had "hot blood" from all the garlic they ate. Japan is another country where garlic is not popular.

Whether you like it or hate it, garlic appears to be an exceptionally good herb that has stood the test of time.

CHAPTER 2

The Versatility of Garlic

Garlic is called a "cure-all" and a "wonder herb." Garlic is very versatile. It is best known for its use in protecting the cardiovascular system. Some people use garlic every day. It is very useful if you feel a cold or a sore throat coming on. Historically, garlic was used for both culinary and medicinal purposes, especially in the Mediterranean areas.

Garlic comes in second to Echinacea in sales on the U.S. Market. Garlic is a member of the lily family and is rich in sulfur compounds. These sulfur compounds give garlic its odor. They also give garlic its health enhancing benefits.

Over a thousand studies, both human and animal, have been done on garlic. Most of these studies seem to indicate that garlic is a powerful ally in the prevention of disease and promotion of good health.

Garlic is credited by research studies as showing promise with improving cholesterol levels, lowering blood pressure, inhibiting blood clots and improving circulation. Studies also show that it is useful for detoxification of the liver and building up the immune system.

Garlic has properties that have a scientific basis. Some researchers think that the allicin that garlic contains is antibacterial and like weak penicillin. Garlic was used during both World War I and World War II when there was a shortage of drugs[2].

Garlic contains antioxidants, which help destroy free radicals. Antioxidants are substances that neutralize free radicals and may help to prevent some of the damage that free radicals can cause. Free radicals are particles that can damage cell membranes and DNA. They may contribute to the aging process and a number of other conditions, including heart disease and cancer.

Garlic contains a number of sulfur-containing compounds that include thiosulfinates, sulfoxides, and dithiins. When garlic is crushed, or chewed these compounds are activated by oxygen and become therapeutic. Allicin seems to be the most potent compound in garlic.

Garlic has antibacterial, antifungal, anti- parasitic and antiviral properties[3]. It is often used for colds, flu, bronchitis, inflammation, athlete's foot and urinary tract infections. It has been used to expel worms from the

---

[2]http://www.med.nyu.edu/content?ChunkIID=21729

[3]http://www.nutrition-and-you.com/garlic.html

intestines. Several studies seem to indicate that garlic can reduce stomach and colon cancer risk[4].

In the area of nutrition, garlic has many nutrients. Among them are manganese, vitamin C, phosphorus, selenium, calcium, potassium, copper, iron, and vitamins B1, and B6. Garlic contains over 200 compounds that include vitamins, trace minerals, flavonoids, and enzymes[5].

More and more researchers are beginning to think that inflammation and oxidation are the underlying causes of many of our chronic diseases. These include high blood pressure, heart and circulation problems, arthritis, cancer and obesity. Garlic has anti-inflammatory properties that can help with all of these conditions[6].

Garlic slows cellular decay, slightly thins the blood and prevents infections. The anti-inflammatory action of garlic makes it a treatment for minor aches and pains. The sulfur substances that Garlic contains are anti-inflammatory enzymes. A study done in 2010 shows evidence that garlic can help to prevent osteoarthritis[7].

---

[4]http://www.webmd.com/vitamins-supplements/ingredientmono-300-garlic.aspx?activeingredientid=300&activeingredientname=garlic

[5]http://www.whfoods.com/genpage.php?tname=foodspice&dbid=60
http://www.nutrition-and-you.com/garlic.html

[6]http://www.whfoods.com/genpage.php?tname=foodspice&dbid=60

[7]http://www.ncbi.nlm.nih.gov/pubmed/21143861

Garlic stimulates perspiration and makes you sweat the toxins and bacteria out of your body.

Garlic was used in folk medicine for everything from Candida and athlete's foot to acne. Garlic is thought to neutralize toxins in the liver.

Some research published in 2003 seems to indicate that allicin, the active ingredient in garlic, may be useful in the fight against potentially fatal infections caught in the hospital[8]. Meanwhile, results of another study revealed that people who took a daily allicin-containing garlic supplement were approximately 50% less likely to catch a cold. Furthermore, those taking the supplement, who did catch a cold tended to recover much more quickly and were significantly less likely to become re-infected[9].

Garlic has traditionally been used to help get rid of intestinal parasites and fungal infections like thrush.

Garlic can be helpful to people suffering from diabetes. It appears to balance the blood sugar. The vitamin C and allicin that garlic contains stimulates the pancreas to release insulin[10].

---

[8] http://news.bbc.co.uk/2/hi/health/3344325.stm

[9] http://www.naturalnews.com/025461_garlic_colds_flu.html#

[10] http://www.academicjournals.org/article/article1380617303_Phil%20et%20al.pdf

According to Dr. Al Sears, garlic can be used to detox from mercury[11]. There was some research done that shows garlic can be an antidote to lead poisoning and other heavy metal poisons[12].

Garlic has traditionally been used to treat internal and external infections. It was used for disorders of the ears, mouth, skin, stomach, and throat. It can be applied externally to boils, and ulcers. In China and India, it has been used for Cholera, dysentery and washing wounds and ulcers. Another advantage of garlic is that it does not create superbugs like antibiotics do[13].

Garlic is said to be good for your colon. The good bacteria that live there feast on garlic. It makes them multiply and outnumber the bad bacteria by keeping them fed. It also gives you a healthy colon[14].

Garlic has been used for everything imaginable at one time or another.

---

[11]http://www.alsearsmd.com/2011/01/six-steps-to-a-pure-and-clean-body/

[12]http://www.naturalnews.com/039338_mercury_heavy_metals_deto x.html

[13]http://www.naturalnews.com/029701_garlic_superfood.html

[14]http://www.npr.org/blogs/thesalt/2013/11/08/243929866/can-we-eat-our-way-to-a-healthier-microbiome-its-complicated

CHAPTER 3

Garlic and the Cardiovascular System

For centuries, people have used garlic for heart problems. The use of garlic for cardiovascular disease is possibly the most studied herbal interaction on record.

Numerous scientific studies have shown that garlic has a role to play in the prevention of heart disease. Epidemiological studies have shown that people in cultures who eat a lot of garlic have fewer heart attacks.

One thing that can cause blood clots is thick blood. In situations like this people are often put on blood thinners. Garlic seems to work as an anticoagulant. It slightly thins the blood so that it is less likely to clot. This enables the blood to flow smoothly through the arteries, and the blood circulation will increase.

When your blood is thin (but not too thin), blockages in the arteries are less likely to occur. If you have thick blood, garlic might be a good option, but *you must check with your health care provider first.*

Taking garlic along with a prescription blood thinner like Coumaden or Plavix can be dangerous. If you are pregnant or have surgery coming up, you should not use garlic. These are times when you don't want your blood to be too thin.

A study in Germany at the University of Saarland found that garlic preserves the elasticity of blood vessels and capillaries. The use of garlic powder taken internally every day helped to increase microcirculation in the capillaries beneath the skin[15].

Garlic has been used for many conditions of the heart and circulatory system. These include high blood pressure, high cholesterol, heart disease, heart attack and atherosclerosis. Scientific studies show that garlic may slow down the process of atherosclerosis and reduce blood pressure[16].

The conclusions of another study indicated that garlic may slow down atherosclerosis (hardening of the arteries) and lower blood pressure[17]. One study that lasted four years found that people who took 900mg daily of standardized garlic powder were able to slow down

---

[15]http://www.ncbi.nlm.nih.gov/pubmed/1930351

[16]http://umm.edu/health/medical/altmed/herb/garlic

[17]http://jn.nutrition.org/content/136/3/736S.full

the development of atherosclerosis. Earlier studies found that garlic appeared to lower high cholesterol.

Garlic has been proven to reduce high blood pressure and reduce heart attacks by lowering the levels of blood fats including triglycerides and LDL ("bad") cholesterol while raising the levels of HDL ("good") cholesterol. In Germany, garlic supplements are licensed as prescription drugs for the treatment of arteriosclerosis[18].

The Journal of the Royal College of Physicians reported that there seemed to be evidence that garlic reduced the parameters of causes of heart disease. They specifically mentioned the lowering of lipids and fats in the blood[19].

An article published in the Journal of Hypertension showed that taking garlic was good for reducing blood pressure. The trial suggests that aged garlic may be a safe treatment for hypertensive therapy[20].

Studies have shown that garlic, because of its value as a natural blood thinner, can be very useful in the treatment of varicose veins, and blood clots[21]. People suffering from intermittent claudication, (poor circulation in the legs) have found this herb useful.

---

[18]Ibid—

[19]http://www.ncbi.nlm.nih.gov/pmc/articles/PMC3652202/

[20]http://www.ncbi.nlm.nih.gov/pubmed/23169470

[21]http://pennstatehershey.adam.com/content.aspx?productId=107&p id=3 3&gid=0001 73

Garlic sulfides create hydrogen sulfide gas (H2S), which helps to dilate blood vessels. This dilation keeps blood pressure under control. Furthermore, these same sulfur elements assist in iron metabolism and are a powerful protector against oxidative damage and high cholesterol.

In another recent study, Russian researchers determined that garlic's beneficial effects on cardiovascular health could be attributed to both direct actions on the walls of heart arteries and indirect preventive actions at the cellular level. Studies have shown that garlic protects the aorta, and helps keep it flexible, thereby extending life.

People should be aware that eating large amounts of Garlic before surgery or dental procedures is not a good idea. It could cause spontaneous bleeding. People taking blood thinners such as Coumadin, or any drugs meant to treat HIV/AIDS virus should always consult with their doctors before taking any garlic supplement, as it may not work well with these drugs.

CHAPTER 4

Garlic and Cancer

Whenever there is a discussion about natural remedies and cancer, there is much that is controversial. There doesn't seem to be as much research about garlic and cancer as there is for garlic and heart disease. I will discuss some of the evidence we have.

There is some evidence that garlic helps to prevent cancers of the digestive system, which includes the esophagus, stomach, pancreas, kidneys, and colon[22].

We know that a healthy immune system is necessary to fight cancer. Studies in test tubes, with animals, and on humans have determined that garlic can reduce the formation of cancerous cells. This appears to show that garlic is a preventative.

Garlic may help the immune system function more efficiently during times of need such as when a person

---

[22]http://www.cancer.gov/cancertopics/causes-prevention/risk/diet/garlic-fact-sheet

has cancer. The protection that garlic offers seems to be related to the amount of garlic that one takes. The American Institute of Cancer Research suggests the use of garlic in a well-balanced plant-based diet[23].

According to a study in the journal *Cancer Prevention Research* researchers determined that eating raw garlic twice a week could cut in half the risk of developing lung cancer. In this study, researchers in China found that people who consumed raw garlic on a regular basis had a 44% lower risk of getting lung cancer[24].

The Centers for Disease Control and Prevention (CDC) show that long-term smoking is the most common cause of lung cancer. What is interesting about this study is that people who smoked and ate garlic had a rate of lung cancer that was decreased by approximately 30%[25].

Several population studies were conducted in China that focused on garlic consumption and cancer risk. In one study researchers found that frequently consuming garlic, onions and chives appeared to be associated with a reduced esophageal and stomach cancer[26].Another study

---

[23]http://www.medicalnewstoday.com/articles/264599.php

[24]Ibid.

[25]Ibid.

[26]Gao CM, Takezaki T, Ding JH, Li MS, Tajima K. Protective effect of allium vegetables against both esophageal and stomach cancer: A simultaneous case-referent study of a high-epidemic area in Jiangsu Province, China. *Japanese Journal of Cancer Research* 1999; 90(6):614–621.

from China showed that a greater intake of garlic and scallions was associated with a 50% reduction in prostate cancer[27].

An analysis of 7 population studies showed that the higher the amount of raw and cooked garlic consumed, the lower the risk of stomach and colorectal cancer[28]. There appears to be evidence that suggests that increased consumption of garlic may reduce the risk of pancreatic cancer. In the San Francisco Bay Area, a study was done that found the risk of pancreatic cancer was 54% lower in folks who consumed more garlic as compared with those who ate less[29].

A randomized clinical study done in Japan compared the effects of daily high-dose and low-dose intake of aged garlic extract. Participants in the study who had colorectal cancer were evaluated after 6 and 12 months. After 12 months, 67% of the low-intake group developed

---

[27]Setiawan VW, Yu GP, Lu QY, et al. Allium *vegetables and stomach cancer risk in* China. *Asian Pacific Journal of Cancer Prevention* 2005; 6(3):387–395.

[28]Fleischauer AT, Arab L. Garlic, and cancer: A critical review of the epidemiologic literature, *Journal of Nutrition* 2001; 131(3s):1032S–1040S.

[29]Chan JM, Wang F, Holly EA. Vegetable and fruit intake and pancreatic cancer in a population-based case-control study in the San Francisco Bay area. *Cancer Epidemiology Biomarkers & Prevention* 2005; 14(9):2093–2097.

new adenomas, and 47% of the high-intake group developed adenomas[30].

Another small nonrandomized study of people with skin cancers involved the application of garlic to skin tumors. In the study, 21 subjects with basal cell carcinoma applied ajoene, a substance found in garlic, to the skin for one month. This substance markedly decreased the size of 17 tumors and increased tumor size in 3 patients and caused no change in 1 other patient[31].

The National Cancer Institute does not support the use of dietary supplements for preventing cancer, but it does recognize garlic as a vegetable with potential anti-cancer properties.

If you are considering taking garlic as a cancer treatment, *you absolutely must consult your oncologist first.* Reputable authorities agree that there is not enough scientific and clinical evidence to consider garlic as a cure for cancer. The study of garlic and cancer treatment is an area where more research is needed.

---

[30]Tanaka S, Haruma K, Kunihiro M, et al. Effects of aged garlic extract (AGE) on colorectal adenomas: A double-blinded study. *Hiroshima Journal of Medical Sciences* 2004; 53(3–4):39–45.

[31]Tilli CM, Stavast-Kooy AJ, Vuerstaek JD, et al. The garlic-derived organosulfur component ajoene decreases basal cell carcinoma tumor size by inducing apoptosis. *Archives of Dermatological Research* 2003; 295(3):117–123.

CHAPTER 5

Garlic and Sex

One of the popular claims for garlic is that it has aphrodisiac powers. Ancient civilizations used garlic for boosting sexuality. In Tutankhamen's tomb, there were clay figures of garlic. For Tibetan monks, garlic is forbidden because of its reputation for aphrodisiac action. Garlic had a reputation as an aphrodisiac in Shakespeare's England. It is used in both the Chinese and the Ayurvedic traditions for the treatment of sexual problems.

The aphrodisiac properties of garlic are considered useful in folklore as a sex rejuvenator. It benefits libido for both men and women[32].

Garlic is reputed to be good for sexual stamina, and it has a reputation for being useful for men who have impotence and prostate problems. The allicin in the

---

[32]https://www.organicfacts.net/health-benefits/herbs-and-spices/health-benefits-of-garlic.html

garlic increases blood flow and dilates blood vessels[33]. The allicin provides more blood flow to the penis.

Garlic aids in blood circulation, which keeps the veins and arteries from aging too quickly. It also helps stimulate nitric oxide, which is required to have an erection.

Garlic tends to normalize blood flow through the penis. The general recommendation is that garlic be taken in the form of 3-4 cloves of garlic a day. After the garlic starts working, one can drop down to three times a week[34].

There is the odor problem with garlic, but if the cloves are crushed and fried in butter, the garlic may still be useful as an aphrodisiac. Frying it in butter may mute the odor somewhat and make it more acceptable to one's partner. The remedy does not always work right away, and you may have to take it for a month before you see results.

If you or your partner just can't handle raw garlic you can get garlic capsules. Some brands have the odor and some brands do not. The allicin in garlic is what moves the blood through the sex organs.

Erectile Dysfunction can mean a man has hardening of the arteries. Garlic is good for this because of its ability

---

[33]http://www.express.co.uk/life-style/health/528133/Superfood-garlic-health-benefits

[34]https://knowyourlove.wordpress.com/garlic-for-sexual-health-stamina/

to boost blood circulation. Men who have heart disease may have impotence problems due to poor circulation and narrowing of the arteries in the groin. Garlic increases the flow of blood to the groin and increases virility.

What about women? Historically garlic is said to be good for women's libido as well as men's. Again it is a matter of blood flow. The garlic increases the flow of blood to the female sex organs and thereby aids in having a positive sexual experience[35].

If you and your partner just can't handle the garlic, don't despair. There are plenty of other herbs, spices and foods that are good for the libido and other sexual problems.

[35]https://www.hersolution.com/info/do-you-know-how-to-increase-sex-drive-in-women-with-spices/

CHAPTER 6

Garlic and Ageing

Ageing is a process that we all have to face. With new breakthroughs in medicine and better sanitation conditions, life expectancy has improved. But along with the length of life comes chronic diseases. One needs to consider the quality of those extra years. Spending your later years in a nursing home is not pleasant. Fortunately, there are things that can make those years more pleasant and give individuals a better quality of life.

There are herbal supplements and formulas that can be helpful in slowing down the ageing process. Garlic is one of them. Ageing is a process that often lowers immunity. Many older people tend to catch more infections and get sick often. Most infections are caused by bacteria, inflammation and viruses.

Garlic fights bacteria, viruses, and inflammation. This makes garlic useful for boosting immunity. Garlic is an anti-ageing remedy that belongs in every older person's health regimen. Some folks believe you can reverse aging by eating one clove of garlic a day. Other folks eat 3 or 4 cloves a day and swear by it. Some folks prefer to take the supplements.

It is true that garlic has that annoying odor, but there doesn't seem to be anything that beats the health benefits of taking the garlic raw.

There are things you can eat with the garlic like parsley, green beans, and apples that mitigate the smell of the garlic. There are garlic supplements on the market that are deodorized. They work well, but if you want what works best go for the raw garlic.

There has been considerable research on Garlic done in the last ten years. Garlic is an antioxidant, and some researchers think garlic can prevent cardiovascular disease, cancer, arthritis, and cataract formation. It can improve circulation and energy levels[36]. These are all problems that plague older folks. Some researchers believe the regular consumption of garlic can reverse ageing.

Garlic has antioxidant properties, and these appear to be useful for slowing the ageing of the liver. It also helps combat the harmful effects of smoking.

Garlic is anti-fungal and can help with yeast infections like *Candida albicans*. It is also effective against intestinal parasites. It seems that researchers are continually

---

[36]http://www.webmd.com/vitamins-supplements/ingredientmono-300-garlic.aspx?activeingredientid=300&activeingredientname=garlic

discovering new uses for garlic in addressing many common medical problems.

There are substances in garlic that enhance one's immune function. Garlic is useful for respiratory illnesses and colds. Garlic is thought to help prevent the formation of cholesterol. The antioxidants in garlic help to prevent hardening of the arteries. These antioxidants can keep your heart healthy and help prevent diseases like atherosclerosis. Garlic also contains nutrients like fiber, Vitamins A, C, E and B-vitamins[37].

Some interesting research was done on garlic and skin ageing. Researchers think wrinkling is caused by too much sun, smoking and stress. The forming of wrinkles is associated with oxidative stress and inflammation. In the study three components of garlic were investigated. The research showed that the components inhibited the breakdown of collagen. The results suggest that garlic had an anti-wrinkle effect due to the anti-oxidant and anti-inflammation properties of the garlic constituents[38].

---

[37] http://www.drheatherkeller.com/wonderfoods/Garlic2.pdf

[38] http://journals.plos.org/plosone/article?id=10.1371/journal.pone.007 3877

CHAPTER 7

Ways to use garlic

According to Dr. Andrew Weil, garlic appears to work best when taken raw. Cooking weakens the antibacterial effects[39].

Eating raw garlic is probably the best way to use it for maximum potency and benefit. Taking two or three cloves in the morning before breakfast is a good way to take it. Good fresh garlic has a bite to it. You can use parsley to counteract the odor, or apples or green beans.

Taking garlic this way is not for everybody. If you just cannot stomach raw garlic, there are many garlic supplements available. I would suggest aged garlic. Another way you can use garlic if you cannot tolerate the taste is to rub it into the soles of your feet. Rubbing your hands with a stainless steel spoon will remove the scent of garlic from your skin.

---

[39] http://www.drweilblog.com/home/2010/7/31/5-reasons-to-eat-garlic.html

In order to benefit from garlic the cloves must be crushed or chopped. Allicin is the component that has most of the health benefits. Allicin does not become active in the clove of garlic until it is pressed, chopped, or crushed and allowed to stand for 10 minutes. The crushing activates the process of converting allin into allicin.

Garlic infusions or teas can be very helpful. Experiment with the various garlic preparations and find the way that it works best for you. I like garlic tea with chicken bouillon and cayenne pepper mixed in. It is great for clearing out your sinuses, and it is also good for colds.

Garlic tea can be combined with many things like ginger, lemon, and pepper. To find good suggestions use one of the search engines on the Internet and do a search for garlic tea.

Garlic is good in winter to help you breathe more easily. It can prevent the flu, colds, and viruses. You can eat raw garlic, or get it in tablets, capsules, and tinctures. Enteric coated tablets help eliminate the odor and have a coating that prevents the destruction of the constituents by stomach acid.

Using Garlic to treat a child for a sinus infection or another ailment is never advised. If your child is sick, call the doctor. It will not hurt your child to have some garlic bread or garlic pizza. Checking with a pediatrician is an absolute must and garlic should never be used to treat your child without professional guidance.

Adults may enjoy some of the great benefits garlic has to offer. Garlic is an herb that can multi-task. It can do several great things for your body. Garlic can help cure and prevent heart disease, high cholesterol, even athlete's foot. Garlic can kill infections whether they are bacterial or fungal.

A sinus infection is painful and awful. Give your doctor a call first, and then consider eating some totally safe garlic. Garlic contains chemicals that kill bacteria, some viruses, and fungal infections. A sinus infection is usually a bacterial infection. Garlic can be eaten raw by adults for optimal infection relief. You can also roast the cloves in the oven to soften their flavor.

Some folks prefer to take their garlic with food. You can chop the cloves raw and add them to sauce or sprinkle them on pasta. You can make garlic bread by buttering some bread and sprinkling garlic powder over it. Pop it in the oven at 350 degrees for five to eight minutes and you have perfect garlic bread. Another idea is to take an ordinary pizza and use the same Garlic powder, available in the spice aisle, to create a tasty garlic pizza.

CHAPTER 8

Remedies

Flea Remedy

According to folk lore, mixing garlic with your dog's food once a day can get rid of fleas. This practice is controversial, and some authorities think that garlic can kill the dog. It might be smart to call the vet before using garlic for your pet.

Homemade Garlic Oil

- Crush cloves of garlic (however much you want to make)
- Cover cloves with olive oil about 1 inch over the garlic
- Let this stand for about three days, shaking daily.
- Strain the garlic from the oil with a coffee filter, cheesecloth or clean white cotton t-shirt.
- Store oil in a jar

How can you use garlic oil? You can use it in cooking for drizzling or frying. You can also use it for ear aches & infections!

Garlic and Honey for Rheumatism

A clove or two of garlic, peeled and then pounded with honey and taken two or three nights successively, is an old-fashioned remedy that is used for arthritis.

Four Thieves Vinegar

There is a famous story about the middle ages when four thieves robbed victims of the bubonic plague and did not seem to get the plague themselves. This was attributed to their consumption of a garlic formula. There is some variation of the various ingredients that were used. Here is one version of the recipe:

Vinegar of the four thieves

- 3 pints of strong white wine vinegar
- A handful each of wormwood, meadowsweet, juniper berries, wild marjoram and sage
- 50 cloves of garlic
- 2 ounces of elecampane root
- 2 ounces of angelica
- 2 ounces of rosemary
- 2 ounces of horehound
- 3g camphor

Steep the plants in the vinegar for ten days. Force through a sieve. Add the camphor dissolved in the acetic acid, and then filter.

Garlic with Chicken soup for Colds and Flu

Take chicken soup, homemade is best, or you can use chicken broth and add fresh garlic to it. You can also add parsley. This remedy is great for colds and flu.

Garlic and Onion Juice for Colds and Flu

Cut thin slices of onion and garlic and cover them with honey. Cover the slices and leave then overnight. During the night, the juice is formed and you should take one teaspoon every 1-2 hours.

Garlic, Lemon and Honey Elixir

This recipe comes from the ancient Tibetans who used it for anti-ageing.

Chop up five heads of garlic and mix with ½ kg of honey. Add the juice of 5 lemons. Pour the mixture into a glass container and cover. Leave it for 8-10 days. Take one tablespoon two times a day before meals.

Garlic oil

Garlic oil can be purchased as oil or in capsules, or you can make your own. Here is one quick way to make up some oil. To make your own, pour some olive oil into a small pot. About one quarter a cup will do. Heat the oil to about 100 degrees. Crush 3-4 cloves of garlic and add them to the oil. Let the mixture cool for 10 minutes.

Strain out the garlic. The oil can be used for earaches, or dabbed onto an insect bite.

Garlic Foot Rub

Here is a remedy you can use if you just can't take garlic orally. Rub garlic oil on the soles of your feet before going to bed. You might want to put on a pair of socks, so you don't get oil all over the bed. The oil is absorbed into your system and works against the cold, flu or infection you may have.

Garlic Tea

Most people have not heard of garlic tea. I f you put the term garlic tea in a search engine on the internet you will get thousands of hits. Here are some recipes for garlic tea.

Garlic Tea I

- 3 garlic cloves peeled and slightly crushed
- 1 Tsp chicken bouillon
- 1 C boiling water
- Honey to taste as desired

Put ingredients in a cup and steep as long as desired. Add honey to taste.

Garlic Tea II

- 3 garlic cloves peeled and slightly crushed
- 1C boiling water

- Honey or stevia as desired

Mix ingredients in a cup, let steep as long as desired. Sweeten as desired.

Garlic Tea III

- 3 garlic cloves peeled and slightly crushed
- 1 bag lemon tea or 1 tsp lemon juice, whichever you want
- 1 C boiling water
- Honey or Stevia

Put ingredients in a cup and steep as long as desired. Add Stevia or honey to taste.

Garlic Tincture

To make a garlic tincture, take 1/8 pound of peeled garlic cloves and put the cloves in 1 cup of brandy. Put in a glass container and seal it tightly. Shake it daily. After two weeks strain it and bottle it. Get a dropper or use a dropper bottle. Take 25-30 drops daily, or as needed.

Garlic for Earache

For an earache, slice a garlic clove. Heat it for a couple of minutes in virgin olive oil and then let it cool. Strain the mixture. Use 1-2 drops in the affected ear.

Garlic and Ginger for sinus infections

Garlic and ginger can be used together in either their raw state or in supplement form. These herbs have anti-inflammatory and antibacterial properties that can help kill bacteria and reduce the swelling in the sinuses or the bronchial tubes.

One way to make this remedy is to make a cup of lemon tea and add some minced garlic. Another way that is perhaps easier is to take supplements of ginger and garlic together. It is easier on the taste buds and the nose since garlic supplements often are deodorized so that they don't have the odor.

CHAPTER 9

Dosages and Contraindications

Garlic Precautions

Garlic and some medications do not mix well. If you are taking medications, you need to discuss using garlic with your health care provider. Garlic slightly thins the blood and when combined with a blood thinning-medication it can cause excessive bleeding.

If you are on Coumadin or Plavix or any other blood thinner do not take garlic because it will cause excessive bleeding. If you are going to have surgery or have a tooth pulled stop using garlic at least 2 weeks prior to surgery or dental extractions to prevent excessive bleeding.

Pregnant or nursing moms should not take more garlic than what is used in food. Garlic can be a stomach irritant if taken on an empty stomach. Liver and kidney damage can occur with excessive use, and topical use can cause blistering and dermatitis. Some people are allergic to garlic, and it can cause light-headedness, vomiting, and diarrhea.

Other common side effects are body odor and bad breath. There may be a burning in the mouth and esophagus. Taking water with the garlic sometimes helps, also just taking less garlic.

Be careful about giving garlic supplements to children. There is very little research on how it affects them or what dosages to give. Consult your pediatrician before using it for a child.

Some other medications that garlic may interfere with are NSAIDS (Ibuprofen, acetaminophen, naproxen sodium, Aspirin), HIV medications and birth control pills.

Garlic used in cooking is usually ok if you avoid massive quantities.

Recommended dosages for adults are as follows:

- 1 or 2 garlic cloves per day, or 2-4 grams a day of minced garlic.
- Aged garlic 600-1200 mg, daily in divided doses
- Tablets: 200mg, 2 or 3 times daily, standardized to 1.3% alliin or 0.6% allicin.
- Fluid extract (1:1 w/v): 4 ml, daily
- Tincture (1:5 w/v): 20 ml, daily
- Oil: 0.03 - 0.12 ml, 3 times daily

About the Author

To contact the author go to:
www.valerielull923@gmail.com

To see the author's website go to:
http://www.valerielull.com

To see the author's blog go to:
simplewaystostayhealthy.wordpress.com

To order additional copies of this book go to:
http://www.valerielull.com
http://www.amazon.com

Other books by Valerie Lull
Ten Healthy Teas
Ten Spices for Health and Longevity

If you enjoyed this book,
please leave a review on Amazon

www.ingramcontent.com/pod-product-compliance
Lightning Source LLC
Chambersburg PA
CBHW061804280526
45787CB00003BA/1474